# PLANT BASED
# INTERMITTENT FASTING

*The Secret to Long-Lasting Weight Loss*

By

Andrea J. Clark

## Copyright © 2017 by Andrea J. Clark

**Disclaimer**

This publication contains the opinions and ideas of its author. It is intended to provide helpful and informative material on the subjects addressed in the publication. It is sold with the understanding that the author and the publisher are not engaged in rendering medical, health, or any other kind of personal or professional services in the book. The reader should consult his or her medical, health or other competent professional before adopting any of the suggestions in this book.

The author and publisher are not responsible for the results that come from the application of the content within this book. This applies to risk, loss, personal or otherwise. This also applies to both direct and indirect application of the information contained within this publication.

Website: http://www.CleanEatingSpirit.com

# Table of Contents

# Introduction

**Is This Book For You?**

You've dieted before. You've lost weight, but gained it back. You've struggled to maintain a healthy body weight. You're overweight, out of shape, but inspired to make a change. You can feel that this time is different, and you want to try something new. You see all these other people who seem to eat what they want, without gaining weight. Well, with this book, you can lose weight, gain energy, and live the life you've always dreamed of. All it takes, is a change of habit.

**The Beautiful Simplicity of Intermittent Fasting**

Dieting and losing weight is hard. If you're reading this book, chances are that you've been disappointed by diets in the past. Weight loss is a very personal journey and it's different for everyone. The mainstream health and fitness world prescribes a one size fits all solution that doesn't fit anyone! In order to lose weight, keep it off, and feel great, we first need to unlearn the lessons of a lifetime, and reteach ourselves the art of intermittent fasting.

What is the "one simple solution" promised by so many professionals? Eat less, and move more. Sounds simple, right? Eat fewer calories, exercise more, and you will lose weight!

We've all tried this at one time or another. At first, it works. You stick it out for a few months, and the weight starts to fall off. Every week you weigh in, and another pound is gone. People have lost tremendous amounts of weight by restricting their calories, weighing their food, and making sure they stay below a certain level of calories.

You try this for four to six months, maybe even a year. You lose 20, 40, even 60 pounds. But at some point, the diet comes to an end. Whether you've reached your goal, or you're just tired of endlessly restricting your calories, it's time to finish that diet and move on to the easier task of weight maintenance.

This is where the problem really shows itself. Despite your best efforts, your continued exercise, and salads for lunch... the weight creeps back on. Pound by pound, you gain back the weight. You tell yourself, if only you'd had more willpower you could've kept the weight off. The truth is, almost everyone gains back the weight.

## The Truth About Calories In Calories Out

What if I told you that it wasn't about willpower? After following that diet of extreme calorie restriction, you are fighting a losing battle against your body. Regaining the weight is not your fault! Why?

After you lose weight through calorie restriction, your metabolism lowers and doesn't go back up. When the diet is over and most of us regain the weight, we feel ashamed and embarrassed that we failed. The truth is, you didn't fail! Regaining the weight after calorie restriction is almost guaranteed. Long-term calorie restriction causes our metabolisms to lower, and our body to use less energy. When we start eating more calories, the metabolism stays low, and the weight comes back on.

## The Solution: Intermittent Fasting

Luckily for you, there is a way to lose weight, regain your health, and increase your overall energy levels without eating an extreme calorie restricted diet. As with any lifestyle change, you need to have willpower, determination, and patience. However, if you put in the work, you'll be more energetic, lose weight, and have a higher metabolism than when you started! What is this mystery program? It's called Intermittent Fasting, and it's about to take the dieting world by storm.

Intermittent fasting is one of the simplest, easiest, and most effective diet plans to follow. Why? Because it isn't a diet plan at all! Intermittent fasting is a pattern of eating. It is a habit that you can easily integrate into your life. This simple change of habit will have incredible effects on your wellbeing and your wallet. You'll feel healthier, live longer, and save money!

Over the next few chapters, we will go over four different methods for integrating intermittent fasting into your life. You'll learn, step by step, how to integrate these styles in your daily routine. By the end of the book, you'll come away with a deeper understanding of what intermittent fasting is, how it works, and why it's right for you.

Whether you're more drawn to the 16/8 plan, eat stop eat, alternate day fasts, or 5/2 fasting, you'll learn all the details, and be able to create the intermittent fasting program that perfectly suits your unique lifestyle.

By changing one small thing about your life, you'll find yourself happier, with more free time, and more money! That's right, this diet program actually saves you money. Through intermittent fasting you will unconsciously eat less, buy less groceries, and spend less money on food.

On top of that, you can practice intermittent fasting anywhere. When you're traveling, busy with work, or strapped for cash, you can always practice intermittent fasting.

What about exercise? Of course, as with any program, exercise is important. On low-calorie diets, people find themselves getting tired more easily, with no energy for intense workouts. With intermittent fasting, the opposite will happen. This eating program causes your body to produce more adrenaline and noradrenaline, giving you boosted energy and motivation to hit the gym.

What foods work best in this new lifestyle change? The best diet is one that works for you long term. The best long-term diet is one that allows for delicious meals, decadent treats, and is good for the planet. In the later chapters, we are going to introduce the basic concepts of the plant-based vegetarian diet, and give you some tips for getting started as a vegetarian.

By switching to a plant based diet, people report cleaner skin, smoother digestion, weight loss, and improved health. By combining the power of a plant-based diet with the simple elegance of intermittent fasting, you'll be on your way to having the fit, healthy, and happy lifestyle of your dreams.

A small caveat before we begin: any diet or weight loss program should be accompanied by exercise. Not only because exercise helps you lose weight, but also because it boost your mood, gives you more energy, and increases your longevity. Begin with a level of exercise that is appropriate for your age and fitness level, and choose movements that you love and can stick with over the long term.

Now, let's learn about the life changing art of intermittent fasting.

# Chapter 1

# What is Intermittent Fasting and Why Does It Work?

Intermittent Fasting (IF) may just be the best-kept secret of the diet and fitness industry. With over 100 years of research to back up this amazing game changing lifestyle, intermittent fasting is poised to take the health and wellness community by storm.

Before we jump into what intermittent fasting is, and why it works, let's first go over a couple of things that intermittent fasting is not.

First, intermittent fasting is NOT a diet plan. There are no off-limits foods, no meal plans, no meal prepping, and no complicated recipes. In fact, you can practice intermittent fasting and eat whatever you want. You'll still get some of the benefits. Of course, intermittent fasting works the best when you try to eat more vegetables and whole foods, while eating less processed foods. It isn't necessary, and you can keep having treats without any guilt.

Second, intermittent fasting is NOT a metabolism lowering calorie restriction game. In fact, intermittent fasting can be used to lose weight, maintain weight, or even gain muscle. What does this mean for you? If you like intermittent fasting, and it ends up being a good fit, you can practice it for the rest of your life. It helps you lose weight, of course, but it has so many more benefits than just that.

## Intermittent Fasting: The Basics

Let's get down to it. What is intermittent fasting? In short, intermittent fasting is a pattern of eating that involves periods of fasting, and periods of feasting. If this sounds frightening, don't worry! You've already been practicing the traditional eating pattern for your whole life.

This is what you've probably been taught: breakfast is the most important meal of the day, and you need to eat it about 30 minutes to 1 hour after you wake up. Your day should consist of three large meals, and two snacks. Many of us, especially those following the Standard American Diet (SAD), have been taught to believe this eating pattern is the best for our health.

But what if there was a body of research out there that proved otherwise? What if I told you that by not eating for periods of 16, 24, or even 36 hours, you could lose weight, gain muscle, and boost your energy levels and overall health? Well this is all true, and it's called intermittent fasting.

There are several different methods of intermittent fasting, and you will learn how to incorporate the top four in a later chapter. For now, let's just go over the basics. To practice intermittent fasting, you don't eat for 16+ hours. For most people, that means eating dinner at 7pm, going to sleep, and then not eating again until lunch the next day. Not eating for 16 hours might sound hard, but it becomes a lot easier if you sleep through 8 of those hours!

You may already have practiced intermittent fasting without realizing it. Have you ever woken up late on a weekend, or met a friend for a late brunch around noon? If that is your first meal of the day, you're practicing intermittent fasting.

If your first reaction to this is reluctance, keep reading. Over the next chapters, we will discuss why intermittent fasting is the right lifestyle for you and how you can easily integrate it into your life.

However, you may think to yourself, *I'll be so hungry if I skip breakfast!* We'll get more into this later, but after the first week or two, you really won't feel hungry! Your mind is used to eating in the morning, so for the first week, you will feel hungry. Once your brain learns to wait until lunch for food, that hunger will go away. In many ways, intermittent fasting teaches you to listen to your body more closely.

## The Science Behind The Lifestyle

To convince ourselves that intermittent fasting really is the lifestyle choice for us, let's go over a few of the scientific reasons why intermittent fasting causes weight loss without damaging our metabolism.

The first truth we need to understand is how the chemistry without our bodies dictates our fat loss and storage. Because when we say we want to lose weight, we mean that we want to lose fat. Now, most people follow the "calories in, calories out" method of weight loss. If you eat fewer calories than you burn, you will lose weight. While this is true, researchers have now shown us that it leaves our metabolisms low, and we are almost guaranteed to put the weight back on.

Intermittent Fasting works because it doesn't rely on the calories in, calories out equation to promote weight loss. Instead, intermittent fasting prompts fat loss by lowering our insulin levels. So, how does insulin work?

## Intermittent Fasting and Your Body's Chemistry

Insulin tells our body when it is time to store energy as fat, and when it is time to burn fat as energy. When we eat, our stomach and liver turn food into energy. Some of that energy goes into our blood stream as blood sugar, and we use that immediately. The rest? Stored as fat.

Insulin is a chemical, released by our pancreas when we eat, that tells our body it is time to store fat. So when we don't eat for 16 hours or more, our insulin level goes down significantly, and our body transitions into fat burning mode. So, even if you ate a large dinner the night before, you'll still go into fat burning mode the next morning!

Insulin isn't the only chemical that a fast triggers, however. When we fast for longer than 16 hours, our body produces more human growth hormone (HGH). This fantastic hormone tells our body to burn fat, repair muscle, and even build new muscles! By fasting, you will lose weight and have more energy!

Yet there is even one more reason that intermittent fasting kicks the calories in calories out method of weight loss: when you fast for over 16 hours, your body produces more adrenaline. Adrenaline, in turn, gives your more energy and mental awareness! You'll feel energetic and thoughtful even when you haven't eaten recently.

The combination of these three effects, lower insulin, increased HGH, and increased adrenaline, combine in your body to raise your metabolism, sometimes up to 14% higher than your base rate. This boost in metabolism can lead to some great weight loss results! You will also be reducing your calories somewhat, since you eat fewer meals each day. This slight calorie reduction, plus increased metabolism, will lead to fantastic and long lasting results.

## The Weight Loss Takeaway

* Intermittent Fasting is NOT a diet, it is a pattern of eating involving fasts and feasts.
* During a fast, insulin levels go down, which tells the body to use fat for energy.
* The body also produces more human growth hormone, which heals muscles and burns fat. * Fasting leads to increased adrenaline in the body.

The combination of low insulin, high adrenalin, and increased human growth hormone, plus slightly lower calorie intake, will lead to long lasting weight loss.

There are more reasons to bring intermittent fasting into your life, some that go way beyond simple fat loss. If you want to improve your quality of life, boost your longevity, and prevent diseases in the future, now is the time to bring intermittent fasting into your life.

# Chapter 2

# The Health Benefits of Intermittent Fasting

Intermittent fasting has helped many people lose weight and become the best versions of them. This pattern of eating is not a short-term diet, but a long-term lifestyle. Why? Because it has a whole list of research backed health benefits that go way beyond weight loss.

Do you have complicated medical histories in your family? Maybe you're nervous about diabetes, or heart disease. The fact is, when the body is in fasting mode, you release hormones that tell the cells in your body that it is time to go into repair mode. In this repair mode, the cells can eliminate many of the first signs of disease. By practicing intermittent fasting, we give our cells more time to heal, providing ourselves with increased longevity in our lives.

## Intermittent Fasting and Diabetes

The first health benefit to come from intermittent fasting originates with that little, fat regulating chemical, insulin. Insulin is probably the most famous for its role in causing or preventing the onset of diabetes.

Today, diabetes is not a debilitating disease, as long as it is caught early and dealt with responsibly. As a matter of fact, most people don't need to suffer from diabetes. Adding intermittent fasting to your lifestyle can help prevent the onset of type 2 diabetes.

Type 2 diabetes is the form of the disease that is mostly triggered by an unhealthy diet and lifestyle. The body develops insulin resistance and therefore cannot regulate the amount of sugar in the blood stream.

When we practice intermittent fasting, the body lowers its overall insulin level. Periods of low insulin help us prevent against insulin resistance. In one study conducted on human subjects, blood sugar was reduced up to 6% during a fast. During that same fast, the insulin level in the body was reduced from 20 to 31%!

A further study conducted in rats with diabetes showed that intermittent fasting helped prevent and protect the kidney from damage. This has not yet been tested in humans.

Okay, so intermittent fasting helps prevent diabetes. But what if diabetes isn't a concern for you? No one in your family has ever had diabetes and your diet right now isn't that bad. Okay, fine. What about a much more common and more deadly disease? What about cancer?

**Intermittent Fasting and Cancer**

It's true, intermittent fasting can help prevent and protect the body from developing certain cancers. How? Let's find out.

First, intermittent fasting can reduce oxidative stress and inflammation in the body. *Oxidative stress* is a fancy way of talking about the cell's natural ability to detoxify itself. If this process of detoxification is interrupted or blocked, oxidative stress occurs. Unfortunately, eating a bad diet, or overeating, can lead to increased oxidative stress and inflammation in the body. These two things can lead to cancer.

There have been a few studies that illustrate the relationship between intermittent fasting and reduced oxidative stress and inflammation. If you're trying to prevent or even heal a chronic disease, or cancer, intermittent fasting could be an excellent choice for you.

Okay, but what if you, or someone you love, already has cancer? Based on a study done on human patients, there is some evidence that intermittent fasting can help reduce some of the side effects of chemotherapy!

Probably the most important benefit of intermittent fasting is it's ability to trigger autophagy in the cells. What is *autophagy*? It's a fancy way of saying "repair mode". When we are eating every three hours, cells are constantly reproducing, using the new food to create new cells. Yet when we pause and enter a short fasting period, the cells shift into repair mode.

This repair mode, known as autophagy, is essential for health cellular life in our bodies. Increasing the amount of repair in our bodies can protect us against certain diseases, including cancer, and Alzheimer's.

**Intermittent Fasting and The Brain**

Yes, that's right, IF can even help prevent Alzheimer's. The research on this claim is still rudimentary, but preliminary studies on rats show that intermittent fasting may delay or slow the onset of Alzheimer's. We need more research on human studies before we can make any bolder claims than that, but for now, better safe than sorry, right?

Even if Alzheimer's isn't a concern for you, there are many more benefits to the brain from intermittent fasting. The boost that IF gives to your metabolism also impacts your brain function.

Studies in animals have shown that intermittent fasting reduces brain damage, strokes, and improves mental functioning over time. Maybe eating your Wheaties in the morning isn't so important, after all.

## Intermittent Fasting and The Heart

You may think we are done here. There can't be ANY more health benefits, right? Wrong. There is one more major health benefit to be earned from a lifestyle of intermittent fasting: lowered risk of heart disease.

Today in America, heart disease is a killer. It is one of the leading causes of death among adults, especially among adults struggling with obesity or weight gain.

Good news for American adults. Intermittent fasting has been shown, through animal studies, to improve on many different risk factors related to heart disease. It reduces blood pressure, cholesterol levels, blood triglycerides, inflammation, and blood sugar levels. Really, there can't be a better lifestyle choice out there where heart health is concerned.

## The Takeaway: Intermittent Fasting and Your Health

That's a wrap on the top health benefits of intermittent fasting! Let's recap, shall we?

* IF can prevent and protect against type 2 diabetes by reducing insulin levels and blood sugar levels.
* IF lowers levels of inflammation and oxidative stress within the body.
* IF triggers autophagy, also known as cell repair. Increase cell repair helps prevent and protect against cancer and Alzheimer's
* IF protects against heart disease by lowering five different risk factors.

Yes, this all sounds too good to be true. A simple lifestyle change such as not eating for 16 hours can lead to all of these benefits? Increased health, weight loss, and boosted energy? It seems impossible. There must be a catch. It must lead to binge eating, because you'll be so hungry after the fast! In the next chapter, let's talk about why this lifestyle does not lead to extra weight gain due to binge eating.

# Chapter 3

# Why You Won't Binge on Intermittent Fasting

Binging, or eating far more than you should in one sitting, is the enemy of weight loss. Unfortunately, however, many people struggle against binge eating, and fall prey to it. Especially those who have already been disappointed by a diet in the past.

Reasons for binge eating can be many and varied. It can have an emotional connection, such as depression or anxiety, or be a stress related coping mechanism, or simply a habit, developed over a long time, and one that can be very difficult to break.

For those who have struggled with over-eating in the past, it can be a major concern when deciding whether to being practicing intermittent fasting. The concern is that by fasting for an extended period, you will grow so hungry, you wont be able to stop yourself from binging once you break your fast.

**Intermittent Fasting and Intuition**

While no official studies have been published about this issue, many case studies can be used to help downplay this fear of overeating.

The biggest gift that intermittent fasting can give to the overeater is the chance to listen to our body. We hear this advice all the time, listen to your body and it will tell you when to eat. For many who are overweight, and prone to overeating, we have lost that ability to listen to our bodies. We feel hungry all the time, or once we start eating, we stop listening to our stomachs.

PLANT BASED INTERMITTENT FASTING

But something different starts to happen after a week or two of intermittent fasting. During your 16-hour fasts, you will get hungry, especially during the first weeks. You will feel hungry during breakfast time, but you can resist it. Then something fascinating happens. A little after breakfast time, the hunger goes away. Even though you didn't eat breakfast, you don't feel hungry any more!

So you go on with your morning, but in a few hours, the hunger comes back. It is stronger this time, but definitely manageable. You wait until your lunch break, and then head out for lunch. This is the first moment of truth. Will your sandwich and salad satisfy you, or will you be driven to over eat?

What many people report, is being able to actually feel satisfied on less food than they were eating before. Why? Because you have learned to listen to your body, to actually feel the hunger, and so you can also feel when the hunger has subsided.

**Intermittent Fasting and Willpower**

The truth is complicated. Intermittent fasting will take some amount of willpower in the beginning. You will have to work hard to skip breakfast, or endure one 24 hour fast. But over time, your willpower will get stronger. Willpower is like a muscle, we only have a limited amount of willpower strength, but we can gain more through practice.

Consider your journey into intermittent fasting like an exercise for your willpower, and your intuition. Although it will be a challenge at first, through this lifestyle, you will increase your overall willpower, and learn how to listen to your body.

This increase in overall willpower can lead to many positive changes in the rest of your life. Increased willpower in eating can also lead to increased willpower towards exercise. Do you have a hard time finding the motivation and energy to go to the gym or stick to a workout plan? With intermittent fasting, you'll have boosted energy, and boosted willpower. Just think of the possibilities!

Now is the time to remind yourself that big changes take time. Intermittent fasting is not a quick fix! Yes, if you follow the plan, you will see results within the first 3 weeks. However, if you want real lasting change, to your weight, your health, and your lifestyle, you will need to be patient. Promise to give IF at least 2 months, and then you can check back in to see just how far you've come.

## The Takeaway

* Intermittent fasting can actually make it easier to listen to your body and eat intuitively.
* By exercising our willpower, we can prevent binge eating.
* With increased willpower relating to food, we can also increase our willpower in other areas of our life, such as work or exercise.

Once you've made the commitment to try out the lifestyle of Intermittent Fasting for 2 months, you may be wondering: how can I get the most out of it? What are the foods I should be eating in order to see the biggest benefit to my health? This is where the plant-based, vegetarian diet comes in. Keep reading to find out why this particular diet can boost your mood, your physical and mental health, and as a bonus, help heal the planet as well.

# Chapter 4

# The Vegetarian Diet: Health and Planetary Benefits

Seen as an unconventional diet for many years, vegetarianism has recently been gaining in popularity, both because of its benefits to human health, and because of its benefits for the planet.

Vegetarianism can bring many benefits to your health and wellbeing. It can improve your skin, digestion, mood, and mental health. It can help reduce carbon emissions and promote local industry. But perhaps even once you've learned all of this, you still feel that you are not ready to commit to being 100% vegetarian.

Well, good news! You don't have to be a vegetarian 24/7, 365 days a year to get the benefits. That's right, you can start with "meatless Mondays" and still eat your normal diet 6 days a week. Or maybe you can commit to trying vegetarian food 3 or 4 days a week. Whatever you choose, even if it's just one day, you will find yourself feeling the benefits. The most important thing is to be patient and fully commit for two or more months.

**The Importance of Protein**

The most important thing to remember when embarking on a vegetarian diet is protein. Many meat eaters make the mistake of removing meat from their traditional meals, and calling it vegetarian. Let's say that you normally love eating steak and potatoes for dinner. Well, sorry to break it to you, but a plate of potatoes is not a well-rounded, nutritious meal.

Luckily for us, there are plenty of readily available plant based proteins on the market today. Soy is the most complete protein, but some people do have allergies to this product. Other proteins include nuts, beans, legumes, and soy based products like tofu and tempeh. Get creative! You'll never find out which vegetarian protein is your favorite unless you try them all!

## A Well Balanced Vegetarian Plate

A good vegetarian meal is made up of three parts: a complex carbohydrate, such as sweet potato, a big pile of veggies, and a delicious vegetarian protein. Adding a healthy fat to some meals will help you ensure a well-rounded diet. Healthy fats are all unsaturated fats, such as nut oils, avocado, flax seeds, and the saturated fat that comes from coconut.

Now that we've got the basics down, let's go over the top benefits of the vegetarian diet for you and the planet. To be clear, we are discussing what is known as *lacto-ovo vegetarian*, meaning a diet including eggs, dairy, and all things vegetarian. Even if you hope to someday become a full vegan, this is a good place to start, as it reduces the changes of nutrient deficiencies.

## Health Benefits: Vegetarian Hearts

The top three medically researched benefits of the vegetarian diet are heart disease, cancer, and type 2 diabetes. Sound familiar? These are three diseases that intermittent fasting can also help prevent! The pairing of plant based intermittent fasting is becoming more appealing by the moment.

Let's begin with the heart. The vegetarian diet is full of "heart healthy" foods, especially grains and legumes. Heart healthy foods are foods high in fiber. Fiber is naturally occurring in all plant-based foods, so naturally the fiber in your diet will increase when you eat vegetarian. For your heart, a diet rich in fiber will reduce cholesterol, and keep blood sugar levels low.

But there is more to having a high fiber diet than heart protection. High fiber diets are also beneficial for the digestive system. Ever have problems with constipation, diarrhea, or digestive discomfort? You can say goodbye to those problems on a well-balanced, nutritious vegetarian diet. The high fiber content, coupled with a decent amount of water, will vastly improve the digestive system.

**Vegetarian Diet and Cancer**

Okay, but what about that dreaded disease, cancer? How does a vegetarian diet help prevent or protect against cancer?

A vegetarian diet mainly consists of fruits and vegetables. The healing properties of fruits and vegetables have long been celebrated, especially where cancer is concerned. These foods are very high in nutrients and minerals, but lower in calories. Berries, for example, are high in anti-oxidants, compounds well known for their ability to fight oxidation in the body. And oxidation can lead to cancer. So, by increasing the amount of vegetables and fruits in the diet, you give your body the tools it needs to fight cancer.

On top of that, certain types of meat are thought to lead to cancer in the body. According to Harvard University, you can eliminate a risk factor for colon cancer by taking red meat out of your diet. So, stop eating red meat, replace it with nuts and beans, and you will have better digestion and a lower risk of colon cancer!

**Vegetarian Diet and Diabetes**

There's one more big health benefit of the vegetarian diet, and that's fighting against type 2 diabetes. Controlling your total calories and getting enough exercise are the most important tools for fighting diabetes, but after that? Avoid red meat. A study by Harvard University showed that women who did not eat red meat were at less of a risk of developing type 2 diabetes.

These are the three big health benefits of the vegetarian diet, but there are lots of smaller benefits to be found along the way. For example, the vegetarian diet, one high in fruits and vegetables, will naturally be also high in water content. This increase in water and nutrients will give you clearer skin, healthier hair, and better functioning of all your internal organs.

Different nutrients have different health benefits, so by eating a well-rounded vegetarian diet, you will naturally be getting more nutrients than a diet of processed foods and meat products. This will in turn lead to a whole host of benefits such as improved muscle function, boosted moods, mental clarity, and increased energy. It takes time and patience to feel all these benefits, but they are out there, just waiting for you to feel them.

So, how can you begin to reap all the health benefits of a vegetarian diet? Begin slowly, and take some time to do your research. At the end of this book, you will find a one-week intermittent fasting vegetarian meal plan that you can follow. It should give you an idea what a well-rounded, nutritious vegetarian meal looks like, so you can begin planning for yourself. Do some research and see what's out there. You may be surprised by how many delicious vegetarian meals are out there!

## The Takeaway

* You don't have to be 100% vegetarian to start seeing the benefits.
* A vegetarian diet can help prevent and protect against heart disease, cancer, and diabetes.

# Chapter 5

# IF STYLE OVERVIEW: 16/8 Method

The 16/8 style of Intermittent Fasting is the easiest and least hunger-inducing version of IF to integrate into your life. This method works on its own, or as a stepping-stone towards longer fasts.

To practice 16/8 IF, you simply fast for 16 hours in a day, then eat for an 8 hour window. This is the shortest fast and the longest feasting window of any of the forms of intermittent fasting. So, what would this style look like?

**How To Practice 16/8**

To practice 16/8 style fasting, begin by skipping breakfast. Eat your first meal of the day after 12 noon. Then you can snack as you like, or have another mini-fast before eating dinner between 6-8pm. After 8pm, you are fasting for 16 hours, until noon the next day.

By following this form, most of your fast happens while you are asleep. It is by far the easiest style of IF for beginners. However, there are some challenges when adopting this form of intermittent fasting.

**The Challenges**

The biggest challenge with this style of fasting, especially for those who really love breakfast, is hunger pains during the morning. For the first week or two you will feel hungry during the time when you would normally eat breakfast.

This is due to the way our brains work. When your brain expects to eat at 8am, it sends signals to the stomach saying "hunger time!" But if you let yourself feel hungry, and wait one hour, something very interesting happens. After the normal breakfast time has passed, the hunger fades. Eventually, after one or two weeks, you won't feel hungry at all in the mornings.

If you're choosing intermittent fasting to lose weight, you should also be aware of your diet during the 8-hour fasting window. Yes, you can eat as you like during this time. However, you won't see results if you eat junk food or overeat. It is best to fill your diet up with vegetables and whole foods.

One last warning for women, there has been some evidence that a 16-hour fast can be unhealthy for a woman. Consider breaking your morning fast with a light snack and 10 or 11am, and having only a 14 or 15 hour fast.

**The Takeaway**

* The 16/8 model of intermittent fasting involves fasting for 16 hours, and eating for 8 hours.
* The easiest way to do this is to skip breakfast, and enjoy your first meal at lunch time. Then, be firm with yourself and stop eating after 8pm.
Pro Tip: You can still drink water, coffee, and tea (with no milk or sugar) during the fasts to offset your hunger.

# Chapter 6 IF Style Overview: Alternate Day Fasting

If you're looking to lose a lot of weight, and you already have very strong willpower, then alternate day fasting may be the solution you have been looking for. This method can be a very extreme challenge, but if that is something you are looking for, read on.

## How To Practice Alternate Day Fasting

Alternate Day Fasting involves not eating for a full day, every other day. Or in other words, a typical week of alternate day fasting looks like this: on Monday you don't eat, on Tuesday eat normally, on Wednesday you don't eat, on Thursday you eat normally, and so on.

Some forms of this diet allow you to eat up to 500 calories on your fasting days, but no more than that. On the non-fasting days, you can eat a normal diet. But as with any other form of intermittent fasting, it is the most effective if you commit yourself to a healthy diet rich in vegetables, fruits, and whole grains.

As with all other methods of intermittent fasting, you are allowed to drink water, coffee, or tea during your fasts, but no milk or sugar.

## Pros and Cons of Alternate Day Intermittent Fasting

This method has been shown to have great health benefits in many of the studies done on intermittent fasting. It will lower your blood sugar, increase insulin sensitivity, and reduce your risk of many diseases.

That being said, this method is quite challenging and may be unsustainable over the long term. If you've been dieting or practicing an alternate form of intermittent fasting for a few weeks or months, then you can think about attempting this form of IF.

For those of you who are significantly overweight, and who have strong willpower and are okay feeling very hungry for half of your days, alternate day fasting can be a great way to lose weight rapidly.

**The Takeaway**

* Alternate Day fasting involves not eating on every other day.
* This is a highly effectively yet challenging form of intermittent fasting.
* Most of the evidence found for health benefits of intermittent fasting was found studying this form of the diet.

# Chapter 7

# IF Style Overview: Eat Stop Eat

Eat Stop Eat is quickly becoming the most popular form of IF within the fasting community. Why? Because its easy, requires little effort, saves you money, and is proven to be effective.

## How To Practice Eat Stop Eat

Eat Stop Eat is quite simple, really. You choose two days of the week, preferably not in a row, and take a 24-hour fast. Now, the important thing to notice here is the difference between the 24-hour fast and the full day fast from the alternate day diet.

Fasting for a full day means that you don't eat at all during that day, waiting a full 36 hours before eating again. But with a 24 hour fast, the fasting window is a bit shorter. So, what would it look like in a real life example?

On Monday, you eat normally. You have an early dinner and finish eating by 7pm. Now your fast begins. Wake up Tuesday morning and fast all day, until 7pm. At 7pm, you can have dinner. This is considerably easier, both physically and mentally, than a full 36 hour fast. You can keep your 24-hour fast from any point in the day, so breakfast to breakfast, lunch to lunch, or dinner to dinner. It doesn't matter as long as you wait the full 24 hours. And of course, water, coffee, and tea are all allowed during the fast, but no milk or sugar.

## The Pros and Cons of Eat Stop Eat

On a positive note, the eat stop eat method is considerably easier than the alternate day fasting model, but slightly more difficult than 16/8. If you've been practicing 16/8 for a period and want to kick up your weight loss, consider adding a few days of 24-hour fasts to your schedule.

Another thing to keep in mind is your exercise routine during eat stop eat fasting. Exercising during a 24 hour fast may be difficult, and many people recommend taking a 24-hour fast during your rest days.

However, if you are eating a low carb diet such as a Ketogenic diet, and your body is using fat for energy, you may still feel high energy during your fast days. If this is the case, consider exercising just before you break your fast. In that way, you will give your body the fuel it needs to repair and rebuild muscle after the workout.

Aside from the mental challenge of getting through a 24-hour fast, there aren't too many downsides to this method. Make sure you eat a normal healthy diet during your eating periods. The big problem can come from binge eating when you finally make it to your next meal after the 24-hour fast. Use your willpower and make sure to eat normally. Do this, and you will see weight loss results.

## The Takeaway

* Eat Stop Eat involves taking two 24-hour fasts in each week, on non-consecutive days.
* A 24-hour fast is different from a 36-hour fast, so you can eat one meal in a day.
* This program is a great next step up from the 16/8 method if you are looking to kick start your weight loss into high gear.

# Chapter 8

# IF Style Overview: 5/2 Diet

This style is perfect for those who are interested in trying 24 or 36 hour fasts, but who are nervous about going without food for that length of time. Though the 5/2 method of IF, you can reduce some of the stress associated with fasting by having small amounts of food during the fast.

## How To Practice 5/2

The 5/2 method is a somewhat simpler method of fasting that can be used on its own, or as a stepping stone to more intense versions of intermittent fasting. So, how does this method work? You eat a normal diet for 5 days of the week, then for two days of the week you restrict your caloric intake down to 500-600 calories.

How would this work in practice? Mondays and Thursday you could eat two small meals of 300 calories or less. Every other day of the week you would eat normally. Wake up on Monday and eat a two-egg omelette with some veggies and cheese, then wait until after work and have a salad with a nice dressing. Sounds doable, right?

## Pros and Cons of the 5/2 Method

The major con of the 5/2 method is the fact that it has never been validated through research. Because you are eating a small amount during the fasting days, there is uncertainty whether your body still registers this day as a fast. However, you could choose to eat your

500 calories at the beginning or end of the day, and then there would still be a significant fasting period involved.

The major pro of this method is the idea of being able to eat a small amount during your fasts. This eliminates a lot of the mental stress associated with fasting. A solid suggestion for beginners looking to graduate to 24 hour or longer fasts is to begin with this method. The 500 calories let your mind adjust to the trial of extended fasting

**The Takeaway**
* The 5/2 method involves eating normally for 5 days a week, then eating only 500 to 600 calories 2 days a week.
* This method has not been tested or proven through research.
* For people with anxiety about fasting, this can be a good introduction to the concept.

# Getting Started:

# Your First Week Action Plan

Now that you've read this book, you're ready to bring the power of intermittent fasting into your own life. Commit to trying this lifestyle for one to two months and you'll never look back. Intermittent fasting will save you money, save you time, help you lose weight, and boost your energy.

With the combined power of intermittent fasting and a vegetarian diet, you will experience steady, sustained weight loss. Once you've reached your goal weight, you can use both of these tools to effectively and easily maintain your goal weight.

Let's get started with your first week action plan. For the purposes of this guide, we will be following the 16/8 method of intermittent fasting, with a feeding period between noon and 8pm. This should be the easiest method for beginners to integrate into their life.

For dietary purposes, this guide will have exclusively vegetarian meals. However, if vegetarianism is new to you, feel free to eat a meal with meat occasionally. For portion sizes, men should increase slightly, women decrease.

Here it is, your one week action plan:

## Monday

8:00am Breakfast: Coffee or Tea, no milk or sugar
12:00pm Lunch: Rice & Black Beans cooked in chili spices, with tomato & corn salsa and guacamole
3:30pm Snack: Apples and peanut butter
7:00pm Dinner: 2 Egg Omelette with tomato, onion, garlic, spinach, and cheddar cheese

## Tuesday

8:00am Breakfast: Coffee or Tea, no milk or sugar
12:00pm Lunch: Caprese Sandwich (Ciabatta Bread, Tomato, Mozzarella, Basil) with a side salad
3:30pm Snack: Trail Mix
7:00pm Dinner: Hearty Vegetable, Bean, and Potato Stew

## Wednesday

8:00am Breakfast: Coffee or Tea, no milk or sugar
12:00pm Lunch: Vegetarian tacos: beans, rice, cheese, salsa, hot sauce
2:00pm Snack: popcorn
4:00pm Snack: Berries and unsweetened yogurt
7:00pm Dinner: Large Garden Salad

## Thursday

8:00am Breakfast: Coffee or Tea, no milk or sugar
12:00pm Lunch: Veggie Burger with side salad
3:30pm Snack: Cheese and Crackers
7:00pm Dinner: Roasted Root Vegetable Medley with Goat Cheese (Choose from sweet potato, russet potato, carrots, pumpkin, and beetroot)

## Friday

8:00am Breakfast: Coffee or Tea, no milk or sugar
12:00pm Lunch: Avocado Toast & Fruit Salad
3:30pm Snack: Roasted Chickpeas
7:00pm Dinner: Linguini with Sautéed garlic, spinach, and cannellini beans

## Saturday

8:00am Breakfast: Coffee or Tea, no milk or sugar
12:00pm Brunch: Eggs Benedict
3:30pm Snack: Apples and peanut butter
7:00pm Dinner: Chickpea and vegetable Indian-style curry

## Sunday

8:00am Breakfast: Coffee or Tea, no milk or sugar
12:00pm Lunch: Green Lentil Salad with lemony dressing and toast
3:30pm Snack: Roasted sweet potato
7:00pm Dinner: Steamed vegetables and white rice with creamy peanut dressing

## Conclusion: Why You Should Start Plant-Based Intermittent Fasting Today

If you make the decision to put yourself, your health, and your wellbeing first, commit to trying intermittent fasting. After only two weeks, you will already begin to feel the many wonderful benefits that intermittent fasting will bring into your self. If you are ready to sleep better, move faster, lose weight, and bring a glow into your appearance, make the commitment to intermittent fasting.

After only a few weeks of this remarkable diet, your mind will completely adjust to the new eating pattern. Yes, the first two weeks can be a bit challenging. If your mind and body are used to eating breakfast at 8am, you will continue to feel hungry during that time. This hunger will eventually fade. After two weeks of intermittent fasting, your mind will adjust, and you will no longer be plagued by hunger pains during the mornings. During those first two weeks, make sure to be busy during your mornings, so that you have tasks and activities that can distract you from the hunger.

The greatest and most immediate benefit to intermittent fasting is the weight loss. After only two weeks, if you commit to eating health and fasting, you will find your clothes slightly looser. You won't lose 10 pounds in a week, but the weight that you do lose, will stay away. After only two weeks, you will notice a slight change in your body weight. After four weeks, others will start to notice as well. Bring this remarkable eating pattern into your life, and watch the pounds slip away.

Your willpower will also grow stronger after only two weeks of intermittent fasting. It is said that willpower is like a muscle, if you exercise it, it gets stronger. Well, overcoming the hunger during those first two weeks is also an exercise for your willpower. Soon, you will find that increased willpower is impacting other aspects of your life as well. You will be able to cut back on overeating, and going to the gym will be easier as well.

This increased willpower is not simply limited to health and wellness. Do you feel you watch too much TV? Your increase in willpower will help you to cut down on screen time. Did you want to start writing more, or pursuing a new hobby? With increased willpower, now you can dedicate yourself with ease. It may seem far-fetched, but intermittent fasting truly can benefit you in every facet of your life.

Whether you arc hoping foi immediate weight loss, or long term improved health and longevity, there are so many benefits from intermittent fasting. Make the positive choice, and take care of your body, your mind, and your soul. Commit to trying intermittent fasting for two months, and watch the benefits pile up. Within a few weeks, you will feel lighter, have more energy, sleep better, have improved digestion, and the willpower to tackle new obstacles. Make the choice to care for yourself. Choose intermittent fasting.

# Bonus Content:

# 6 Vegetarian Recipes for a Healthier You!

This collection of vegetarian recipes has been especially collected for people who are looking to lose weight and improve their lives using intermittent fasting and a vegetarian diet. The recipes are healthy, well balanced, and full of nutrients without compromising on flavor. Because intermittent fasting eliminates the need for calorie counting, calories are not included per serving, but the portion sizes should be followed for best results.

# Vegetarian Rice & Beans

Rice & Beans is an excellent vegetarian go-to meal for lunch or dinner. Why? Because it's filling, it comes with healthy, unprocessed carbs, and the beans are packed full of protein. You can mix in whatever spices you like. In this recipe, we will use a Mexican inspiration for flavor. This nutrient-packed meal will give you the energy to get through the rest of your day like a champion.

**Ingredients (serves 4)**

- 1 cup brown rice (white if pressed for time)
- 1 can black beans, rinsed and drained
- 3 tablespoons tomato paste
- 1 medium onion, diced
- 1 bell pepper, chopped
- 3 cloves garlic, smashed
- 1/2 teaspoon cumin
- 1/2 teaspoon paprika
- 1/2 teaspoon chili powder
- 1/2 tablespoon olive oil
- 1 lime
- Salt and pepper

## Directions

1. In a large pot, combine 2 1/2 cups of water with all the spices (cumin, paprika, chili powder) and the oil, rice, and tomato paste. Add a dash of salt. Bring to a boil, then allow to simmer. Cook until rice is tender, about 30 minutes.

   * Rice Pro Tip: Always cook rice with a little more than a 2:1 ratio of water to rice.

2. While the rice is cooking, heat up a frying pan and add a splash of oil. Sautee onions, garlic, and bell pepper on medium heat until onions turn translucent. Add black beans and sauté for a further 3 minutes.

3. Mix veggies and beans into the rice. Squeeze lime into the mixture. Let sit for 5 minutes, then serve.

4. Optional: Serve with fresh salsa or guacamole, and wrap it up in lettuce leaves for a fun, taco inspired dish.

# Easy 2-Egg Vegetarian Omelette

Omelettes are a savory, quick, and easy meal that is nutritious and filling. Although initially they can be intimidating to make, and can often turn into "Scramb-omelettes" the first few times, once you get the hang of it, you'll be whipping up omelettes for dinner every week. Nutritionally speaking, the eggs give you heaps of filling protein, with a bonus pack of valuable nutrients, and the veggies add much needed flavor, fiber, and nutrients to get you through to your lunch the next day.

## Ingredients (serves 1)

- 2 Eggs
- 1 tablespoon milk
- 1/4 onion, diced
- 1/2 bell pepper, chopped
- 2 cloves garlic, smashed
- 1/2 cup spinach
- 1 teaspoon olive oil
- 1/4 cup shredded cheddar cheese
- Salt and pepper

## Directions

1. In a small bowl, crack the two eggs, and add the milk and a pinch of salt and pepper. Whip until fully blended. Set aside.
2. Heat a frying pan over medium heat for 2 minutes. Add olive oil, onions, and garlic and sauté until onions begin to turn translucent. Add bell pepper and spinach, sauté for 3 more

minutes, or until spinach is fully wilted. Remove from pan and set aside.

3.  Re-heat the pan, add another splash of olive oil. Reduce heat to medium low, then pour egg mixture into the pan. Cook for 1 minute on medium-low heat.
4.  Sprinkle cheese and black pepper over the egg mixture. Once the eggs are almost fully cooked through, add the veggies on top, then fold in half. Cook for 1 to 2 more minutes.
5.  Remove from pan, let sit for 5 minutes. Enjoy.
6.  Optional: Enjoy with salsa, guacamole, or ketchup.

# Quick Caprese Sandwich

Caprese is one of the simplest and most delicious vegetarian sandwiches on the market. For the carnivore who can't imagine a sandwich without a pile of deli meat wedged in between two slices of bread, it may come as a shock how completely delicious and filling this caprese sandwich is. Take a risk, try this vegetarian sandwich, and allow yourself to be converted to the world of vegetarian sandwiches.

## Ingredients (serves 1)

- Ciabatta roll
- Mozzarella cheese
- 1 tomato, thinly sliced
- Fresh basil
- 2 teaspoons basil pesto
- Olive oil
- Salt & black pepper

## Directions

1. Slice the ciabatta role through the center and drizzle olive oil over the inside of both halves.
2. Spread basil pesto across the bottom half, then layer tomato slices and mozzarella slices on top.
3. Sprinkle salt and black pepper to taste on top of the tomato and mozzarella, then lay some fresh basil leaves on top. Close the sandwich with the top of the bread, and enjoy.
4. Optional: serve with a fresh garden salad with balsamic dressing for a more complete meal.

# Hearty Vegetable Stew

A warm bowl of stew is the perfect meal for cold winter nights or chilly fall days. The flavors in this stew bring together the earthiness of root vegetables, with the brightness of herbs and spices. The filling fiber of the beans makes it a complete dish. Fill up on this delicious stew any night and go to bed happy and healthy.

**Ingredients (serves 4)**
- 2 1/2 cups chopped potatoes
- 1 1/2 cups chopped carrots
- 1 cup chopped celery
- 1 onion, diced
- 4 cloves garlic, diced
- 1 can kidney beans
- 2 cups vegetable broth
- 2 cups water
- 3 tablespoons tomato paste
- 1 tsp thyme
- 1 tsp rosemary
- 1 tsp paprika
- 1/2 tsp cayenne pepper
- Salt and pepper to taste

## Directions

1. Heat a large pot over medium heat for 2 minutes. Pour in the olive oil, then sautee the onion and garlic until the onions become translucent.
2. Pour in the water, broth, spices, and herbs. Stir well, and bring to a boil.
3. Add the potatoes, carrots, celery, and kidney beans. Bring to a simmer. Cover, cook for 20 minutes, or until potatoes and carrots are fully cooked.
4. Remove from heat and let sit at least 10 minutes.
5. Serve with a slice of wholegrain bread, or with a sprinkle of cheddar cheese over the top.

# Gluten-Free Homemade Veggie Burgers

This quick and easy recipe for veggie burgers is the simplest recipe you'll find. Most veggie burger recipes require a long list of beans and vegetables, ample time blending everything and mashing it together, and an overly complicated list of instructions. Instead, these veggie burgers require only 5 ingredients, are easy to put together, and delicious to eat. Enjoy them for lunch, dinner, or as a midday snack.

**Ingredients (serves 6 large patties, 10 small):**

- 4 large potatoes
- 3 carrots
- Up to 3 cups Oat or Chickpea flour (or regular flour)
- 1 tsp Salt
- 1/2 tsp Pepper (or more, to taste)

**Directions**
1. Finely shred the potato and carrots. Mix the vegetables together with the salt and pepper. together in a large bowl. The mixture should be very wet from the moisture of both vegetables.
2. Begin to add the flour. Add 1/2 cup at a time, and mix into the vegetable mixture with your hands. As you add more and more flour, the mixture will naturally begin to bind together. Add flour and mix together until you can easily form patties that don't crumble.
3. Form the dough into vegetable burgers.

# Two Cooking Options:

## Options 1: Frying

1. Heat a pan over medium heat and add oil. The oil should cover the whole pan, but it doesn't need to be deep enough to cover the burgers.
2. When the oil is hot, add the burgers and cook for 4 minutes, or until the bottoms are browned but not burnt.
3. Flip the burgers and cook the same on the other side.
4. Remove the burgers from the pan and let them sit on paper towels to draw out excess oil.

## Option 2: Baking

1. Baking is the healthier option, but can result in drier burgers. Be sure to pat some oil onto the burgers before baking.
2. Heat an oven to 325F
3. Place the burgers into an oven safe pan, with at least 1 inch between each burger.
4. Bake in the oven for 10 minutes, or until the burgers have a solid crust, and are browned but not burnt. Remove from oven and let rest 10 minutes.

Enjoy these burgers in whole grain buns, or in lettuce wraps with your favorite burger toppings!

# Roasted Chickpeas

Roasted chickpeas are the perfect vegetarian snack. You can make them beforehand, they can take on many different flavor combinations depending on what spices you use, and they are crunchy, healthy, and full of protein. How is that for guilt free snacking?

## Ingredients
- 1 can of chickpeas, rinsed and drained
- 1 tsp salt
- 1/2 tablespoon olive oil
- Flavoring of choice
- Suggested flavors: 1/2 teaspoon cumin, Juice of 1/2 lime, black pepper, 1/2 tsp turmeric
- Parmesan cheese, rosemary, salt
- Indian curry powder, salt
- Soy Sauce, Wasabi powder

## Directions
1. Preheat the oven to 350F
2. In a large bowl, mix together the chickpeas, salt, olive oil, and flavorings of choice.
3. Mix together all the ingredients until the chickpeas are evenly coated with flavors.
4. Pour this mixture into a greased oven pan.
5. Bake the chickpeas in the oven for 10 minutes, shaking occasionally to make sure the chickpeas do not stick to the pain.

6. Chickpeas should be hard and crunchy, not soft at all. If the chickpeas are still soft, continue to roast them.

7. Remove from oven and wait 10 minutes before eating. Roasted Chickpeas can be stored in an airtight container for 3 days before going stale. Perfect for midweek snacking!

# Author's Note

Thank you so much for taking the time to read my book. I hope you have enjoyed reading this book as much as I've enjoyed writing it. If you enjoyed this book, please consider leaving a review on Amazon. Your support really means a lot and keeps me going.

If you have any questions, please don't hesitate to contact me at ask@cleaneatingspirit.com
Don't forget to follow me on Facebook and Instagram for more information related to health and wellness.

Facebook: https://www.facebook.com/cleaneatingspirit/
Instagram: https://www.instagram.com/cleaneatingspirit

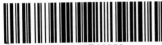
43703945R00030

Made in the USA
Middletown, DE
16 May 2017